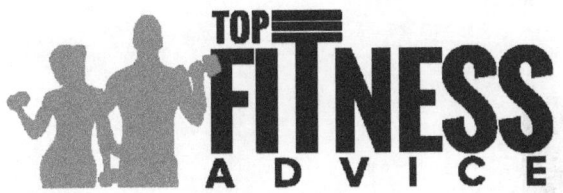

# THE VITAMIN D HEALTH BOOK

*3rd Edition*

Learn Exactly How Vitamin D Can Help With Weight Loss, Healthy Living & Boosted Energy!

**LINDA WESTWOOD**

First published in 2015 by Venture Ink Publishing

Copyright © Top Fitness Advice 2019

All rights reserved.

No part of this book may be reproduced in any form without permission in writing from the author. No part of this publication may be reproduced or transmitted in any form or by any means, mechanic, electronic, photocopying, recording, by any storage or retrieval system, or transmitted by email without the permission in writing from the author and publisher.

Requests to the publisher for permission should be addressed to publishing@ventureink.co

For more information about the contents of this book or questions to the author, please contact Linda Westwood at linda@topfitnessadvice.com

## Disclaimer

This book provides wellness management information in an informative and educational manner only, with information that is general in nature and that is not specific to you, the reader. The contents of this book are intended to assist you and other readers in your personal wellness efforts. Consult your physician regarding the applicability of any information provided in this book to you.

Nothing in this book should be construed as personal advice or diagnosis, and must not be used in this manner. The information provided about conditions is general in nature. This information does not cover all possible uses, actions, precautions, side-effects, or interactions of medicines, or medical procedures. The information in this book should not be considered as complete and does not cover all diseases, ailments, physical conditions, or their treatment.

You should consult with your physician before beginning any exercise, weight loss, or health care program. This book should not be used in place of a call or visit to a competent health-care professional. You should consult a health care professional before adopting any of the suggestions in this book or before drawing inferences from it.

Any decision regarding treatment and medication for your condition should be made with the advice and consultation of a qualified health care professional. If you have, or suspect you have, a health-care problem, then you should immediately contact a qualified health care professional for treatment.

No Warranties: The author and publisher don't guarantee or warrant the quality, accuracy, completeness, timeliness, appropriateness or suitability of the information in this book, or of any product or services referenced in this book.

The information in this book is provided on an "as is" basis and the author and publisher make no representations or warranties of any kind with respect to this information. This book may contain inaccuracies, typographical errors, or other errors.

Liability Disclaimer: The publisher, author, and other parties involved in the creation, production, provision of information, or delivery of this book specifically disclaim any responsibility, and shall not be held liable for any damages, claims, injuries, losses, liabilities, costs, or obligations including any direct, indirect, special, incidental, or consequences damages (collectively known as "Damages") whatsoever and howsoever caused, arising out of, or in connection with the use or misuse of the site and the information contained within it, whether such Damages arise in contract, tort, negligence, equity, statute law, or by way of other legal theory.

# Table of Contents

| | |
|---|---|
| Disclaimer | 3 |
| Introduction | 7 |
| Chapter 1: A Little Bit About Vitamin D | 9 |
| Chapter 2: Source of Vitamin D | 15 |
| Chapter 3: The Various Ways Vitamin D Helps You Lose Weight, Get Healthy, and Increase Your Energy Levels | 19 |
| Chapter 4: What Happens to People Who Have Vitamin D Deficiency? | 37 |
| Conclusion | 43 |
| Final Words | 45 |

# Would you prefer to listen to my book, rather than read it?

# Download the audiobook version for free!

If you go to the special link below and sign up to Audible as a new customer, you can get the audiobook version of my book completely free.

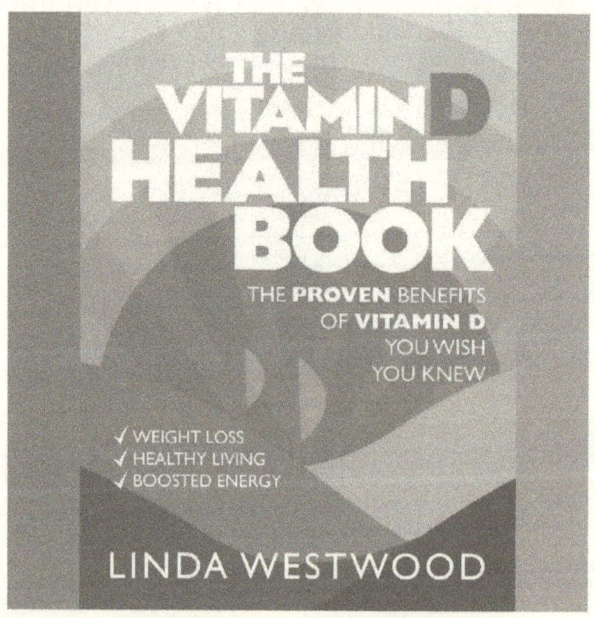

Go here to get your audiobook version for free:

**TopFitnessAdvice.com/go/VitaminD**

# Introduction

Vitamin D is a very unique vitamin different from other types of vitamins. Its uniqueness stems from the fact that it functions both as a vitamin and a hormone.

Vitamin D is one of the most important vitamins needed by the body due to the major role it plays in the body's diverse processes.

The immune system functions better when there is a high level of vitamin D in the blood. It keeps your energy levels very high because of its primary role in improving muscle function. Above all, individuals with adequate amount of vitamin D have less risk of getting overweight.

It is the only type of vitamin our body produces internally, which we get from the direct rays of the sun (the reason why it's also known as the "sunshine vitamin").

However, other types of foods also contain vitamin D, and we can also get it in supplements, making it readily available to anyone. This report is going to look into the different forms of vitamin D, its various benefits, and how we can use and apply them to our general wellbeing.

## Chapter 1

# A Little Bit About Vitamin D

## Vitamin D - Sources and Function

There are three major sources of vitamin D: sunlight, food, and supplements.

Of the three, sunlight is known to be the best source, but it is not regularly available due to seasonal change of weather. When it is received in excess, the sun is known to cause wrinkles, photo-damage, cancer and other problems.

So, the major challenge here would be to find a striking balance between receiving the right level of vitamin D and preventing the adverse effects of the sun on the skin.

## The Sunshine Vitamin

It is important to note that there are four main factors that determine the level of vitamin D you would receive from the sun: the altitude of the earth, latitude, time of year, and hindrances to sun exposure.

Those who stay in higher altitudes will have better exposure to the sun since there are fewer atmospheres that will block the sun rays.

On a similar note, individuals that stay closer to the equator will feel more impact of the sun throughout the day and even throughout the months of the year than those who stay farther than the equator.

Sun rays have more direct impact on the skin during the summer than during winter. This increases the production of vitamin D by the skin.

Another important factor to consider is human and natural impediments to sun exposure. Umbrella, hat, smog, and the cloud hinder the impact of the sun on the skin.

These all reduce the extent of sun exposure, thereby limiting the production of vitamin D in the body. Any factor which lessens the penetration of ultraviolet light on the skin will definitely limit the production of vitamin D.

I hope that you are enjoying this book so far, and if you could spare 30 seconds, I would greatly appreciate you leaving a review on Amazon.com.

# Discover Scientifically-Proven "Shortcuts" & "Hacks" to Lose Weight FASTER (With Very Little Effort)

For this month only, you can get Linda's best-selling & most popular book absolutely free – *Weight Loss Secrets You NEED to Know*.

Get Your FREE Copy Here:
**TopFitnessAdvice.com/Bonus**

Discover scientifically-proven tips to help you lose weight faster and easier than ever before. With this book, readers were able to improve their weight loss results and fitness levels. So, it's highly recommended that you get this book, especially while it's free!

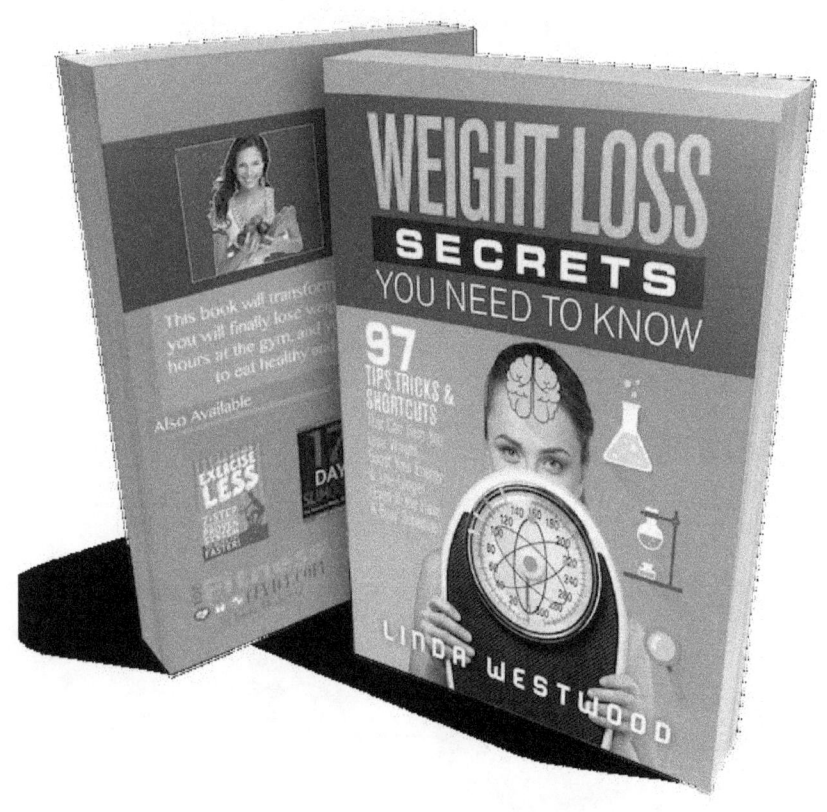

Get Your FREE Copy Here:

**TopFitnessAdvice.com/Bonus**

Chapter 2

# Source of Vitamin D

## Food Sources of Vitamin D

There are basically two main types of food that can give you vitamin D: foods that provide natural vitamins, and foods that are fortified with it during the production process.

Most fortified foods are typically breakfast cereals or milk. There are quite a few foods that contain a considerable amount of vitamin D, which will make them worthwhile to eat when that is your main purpose for eating them.

These sources include some types of orange juice, milk, tuna fish, mackerel, mushrooms, salmon, and cod liver oil. Below are the best foods with the highest concentration of vitamin D.

- **Mushrooms**

    Humans have the ability to produce vitamin D when exposed to the sun rays, and the same is true of mushrooms. But not all mushrooms will contain vitamin D, because most of them are usually grown in the dark and may not see enough sunlight. Certain types are grown in ultraviolet lights to prompt vitamin D production. An example of such mushrooms is Portobello mushrooms. A 3-ounce serving of this mushroom can get you about 450 IUs of vitamin D.

- **Fortified Milk**

This is another great source of vitamin D. Generally, 6 ounces of yogurt contain about 80 IUs of vitamin D, while a glass of milk (8 ounce) contains about 90 IUs. This level can be lower or higher depending on the quantity you add.

- **Fatty Fish**

Common types of fatty fish that can give you vitamin D include eel, tuna, mackerel, trout, and salmon. Usually, about three ounces of salmon can get you 400 IUs of vitamin D. With this meal you will also get an added bonus of Omega fatty acids. Boosting your vitamin D intake does not only have to come from fresh fish. There are also canned fish with good levels of vitamin D. Canned sardines and canned tuna fish both have a considerable level of vitamin D, and they are even less expensive.

- **Vitamin D Supplements**

The constant research and study on the benefits of vitamin D has resulted in a lot of findings regarding the best ways to get vitamin D through supplements. There are vitamin D supplements of various forms, shapes, and sizes. If case you can't get enough of vitamin D from the sun and your diet, you don't need to worry because supplements can provide just enough for you.

There are two basic forms of vitamin D used as supplements: pre-vitamin or ergocalciferol vitamin (or what is most commonly known as vitamin D2) and cholecalciferol (vitamin D3). The latter can equally be produced by the body.

It is important to note that a supplement is always a supplement and may not be used as a replacement or substitute for sunlight. So, you will still need the natural vitamin produced by your body through the direct ultraviolet light of the sun. Moreover, you may not be able to get the right level of vitamin from food alone, so a combination of the three major sources of vitamin D is needed to get the required level needed by the body.

Once again, thank you for reading this book, and I hope you're getting a lot of valuable information. I would greatly appreciate it if you could take 30 seconds to leave me a review for this book on Amazon.com.

# Enjoying this book?

# Check out my other best sellers!

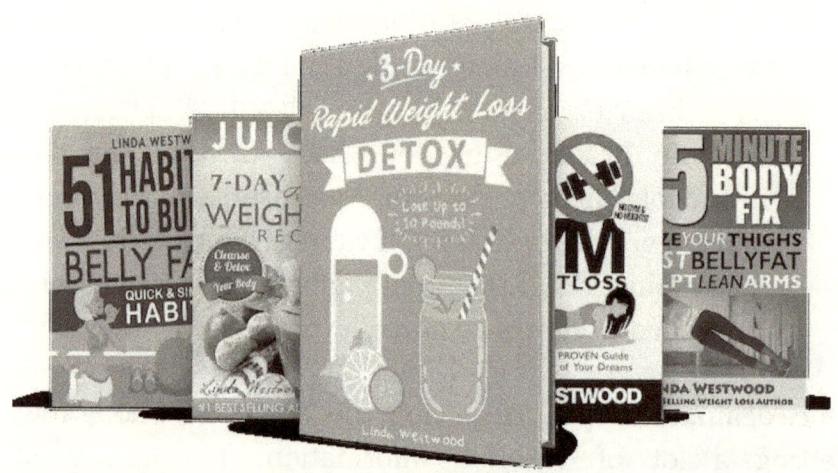

Get your next book on sale here:

**TopFitnessAdvice.com/go/books**

## Chapter 3

# The Various Ways Vitamin D Helps You Lose Weight, Get Healthy, and Increase Your Energy Levels

Now that you are aware of the different ways of getting vitamin D, let's go into the business of the day, which is finding out what it can do for you, and how best to utilize it.

Vitamin D plays a very important role both in your dietary habits and immune system functioning. Below are 28 reasons why you need the right levels of vitamin D in your body.

## 1. Weight Gain Prevention

Research has proven that Vitamin D can prevent weight gain that usually occurs in middle aged women. When there is enough vitamin D in the body, the fat storing behavior of fat cells is greatly reduced. But when there is a low level of Vitamin D in the bloodstream, levels of calcitriol and parathyroid hormone increases, which is really bad. When there is a high level of these hormones in the body, they begin to hoard fat rather than burn it.

Research has it that vitamin D improves fat loss efforts, controls appetite, enhances the immune system, improves serotonin levels, as well as lowers the insulin level in the body.

All these roles contribute to lowering the accumulation of fat in the body. To back this up, a recent study at the University of Minnesota discovered that a greater level of vitamin D at the beginning of a low-calorie diet is known to increase weight loss efforts.

This research discovered that the subjects used for the study ended up shedding almost a pound more on the restricted diet when vitamin D increased in their blood.

## 2. Using Vitamin D for Weight Loss

According to the NIH (National Institute of Health), supplements that contain vitamin D are very effective for weight loss. However, it is much more effective when taken with calcium. Also, taking vitamin D supplements alone might not help you entirely lose weight.

But adding vitamin D supplements with your regular exercise can help an individual speedily reduce their weight. Gloomy pre-spring weather can actually increase fat storage in our body.

Vitamin D is produced by the body when it is exposed to the UVB rays of the sun. Apart from the already known immune benefits, a good level of Vitamin D is known to trigger the production of leptin, a mechanism that helps the body slim down by signaling the stomach and the brain to blunt your appetite.

If you don't have the urge to eat all the time, you will be minimizing the risk of weight gains.

## 3. Health Benefits of Vitamin D for the Common Cold

This benefit of vitamin D may not be known by a lot of people, but studies have shown that there is a relationship between vitamin D and prevention of the common cold. It is not surprising that people tend to get the cold and the flu, mostly during winter when the sun (a main source of vitamin D) has limited presence.

To make this point clearer, there have been recent studies that have linked vitamin D to common cold prevention. One such study is the publication of the Archives of Internal Medicine, where it was discovered that keeping a high level of vitamin D staves off the cold.

The research, which studied about 19,000 people, revealed that people with the lowest levels of vitamin D are more prone to respiratory infection than those with the highest levels of vitamin D.

## 4. Prevention of Chronic Fatigue Syndrome

Vitamin D has long been a major recommended supplement for people suffering from chronic fatigue syndrome. This is also associated with the muscle.

Because vitamin D helps you build strong bones and strong muscle, the risk of developing chronic fatigue syndrome will be greatly minimized. To get vitamin D for this purpose, you have to take enough vitamin supplements as well as adding some foods rich in vitamin D in your daily diet.

## 5. Vitamin D Ensures Healthy Bones

One major role vitamin D plays in the body is the control of calcium and the maintenance of the levels of phosphorus in the blood. These are two basic factors that are necessary for the maintenance of a strong healthy bone. This is why the deficiency of vitamin D in the body causes rickets in children.

When an adult is lacking vitamin D in the body, it can lead to osteoporosis or osteomalacia, which cause muscular weakness and bone density. This is the most frequent bone disease among older women and post-menopausal women.

Maintenance of a high level of vitamin D in the body would drastically reduce the risk of having such problem.

## 6. Reduced Risk of Diabetes

A lot of studies have revealed an inverse relationship between risk of type 2 diabetes and blood concentrations of vitamin D. Inadequate levels of vitamin D may have a negative effect on glucose tolerance and insulin secretion.

When there is an adequate level of vitamin D, the body, tends to produce a balanced level of insulin, which minimizes the risk level of diabetes.

## 7. Healthy Pregnancy

Lack of or inefficient vitamin D in the body is linked to bacterial vaginosis and gestational diabetes mellitus in pregnant women.

Also, pregnant women with vitamin D deficiency, are at greater risk of developing pre-eclampsia and would need a caesarean section. But the presence of high levels of vitamin D in pregnant women helps the mother throughout the pregnancy and during childbirth.

## 8. Prevention of Cancer

A high level of vitamin D in the body is known to help prevent cancer. It is extremely vital for cell-to-cell communication and regulating cell growth.

Research has shown that calcitriol (which is another form of vitamin D) can lessen the progression of cancer by reducing the proliferation of cells, increasing cancer cell death, and slowing the development of blood vessels in cancer tissues.

## 9. Immune Support

The immune system has killer cells that help destroy pathogens and fight foreign attacks on the body. Vitamin D is known to support these cells.

These killer cells stay idle in the body until their service is needed to fight foreign attacks. They will remain dormant in the body until certain reactions in the body activate them.

Vitamin D is one of the most vital hormones that helps activate these cells. Vitamin D supports the activation of these cells and also alerts the cells to go back into dormant state when their job is done.

If these cells are not alerted to fight off invaders, it could lead to autoimmune disorders.

## 10. Provides Protection Against Polycystic Ovarian Syndrome (PCOS)

PCOS is a major cause of infertility among women. People who have this syndrome are Vitamin D deficient.

A recent study conducted in 2011 showed that metabolic risk factor in PCOS women is more prone when there is a deficiency of Vitamin D.

## 11. Helps Fight Different Types of Infections

It is far more effective, less expensive, safer, and even more prudent to increase Vitamin D levels in the body than getting vaccinated against body infection.

Because the immune cells make use of Vitamin D, there is a strong evidence that it will help destroy tuberculosis bacteria.

So, a considerable level of Vitamin D in the body will definitely contribute to fight off different infections caused by bacteria in the body.

## 12. Provides Relief for Depression Symptoms

Some studies have revealed that Vitamin D (especially D3 supplements) may be helpful in treating seasonal affective disorder. Doctors always recommend light therapy for people who are suffering from the seasonal affective disorder.

In most cases the Vitamin D that is created in the body when it is exposed to the sun might not be adequate to get the right level of the vitamin in the body. But taking D3 supplements might ease some of the symptoms linked with depression due to low sunlight during winter.

## 13.     Maintaining Calcium Levels

Calcium is a vital nutrient the body and bones need for proper development. When there is inadequate calcium in the body, it can lead to a series of body disorders, which includes rickets in children.

The production of calcium in the body is enhanced by Vitamin D. When there is a low level of Vitamin D-3, it can result to osteoporosis in aging adults and rickets in babies.

## 14.     Prevention of Influenza

There was a comprehensive research on the patterns of disease complications and deaths during the 1918 influenza pandemic that killed more than 500,000 people.

The research discovered that fewer flu complications and deaths were recorded in the southern cities where there is higher level of sunlight throughout the year.

Contrastingly, the most deaths from the pandemic occurred in the northern cities, where they usually experience less sun exposure.

Although this association may not be conclusive enough to suggest that the cause of this difference was lack of Vitamin D, other research and proofs have certainly supported the claim that a considerable exposure to the sun largely decreases the chances of influenza.

But the underlying fact that Vitamin D can help fight respiratory infections cannot be argued due to mechanisms that support this fact.

La-hydroxylase, an enzyme that converts dormant Vitamin D to its active form, is secreted by long cells, which contribute immensely to fighting respiratory infections.

I hope you have learned something from this book so far and would greatly appreciate it if you could leave an honest review on Amazon.com.

## 15. Improves Muscle Function and Increases Strength

People who always feel weak can ease their discomfort by improving their vitamin D levels in the body.

New studies have shown that vitamin D and muscle function have a close relationship—including recovery from daily activities and exercise. The study also revealed that lower levels of vitamin D can result in physical fatigue.

In a similar study conducted in adolescent girls, it was revealed that vitamin D has a close relationship with velocity, force, and muscle power. So, a high level of this vitamin in the body can greatly increase your muscle function.

## 16. Improves Lung Function

Do you know that vitamin D can contribute immensely in helping you breathe easier?

Yes, new research has revealed that the deficiency of vitamin D is known to cause rapid lung decline and worse lung function in smokers over time.

This study suggested that vitamin D may have a major role in protecting against some side effects of smoking on the lung. Vitamin D is not just a vitamin, but also a hormone that corrects several imbalances in the body.

## 17. Vitamin D Also Helps in the Reduction of Blood Pressure

Hypertension is one of the primary causative factors of high blood pressure.

In 2012, the European Society of Hypertension presented a report that shows how vitamin D supplements can help reduce blood pressure in patients suffering from hypertension.

On a similar note, another study discovered that the deficiency of vitamin D in premenopausal women might add to the risk of the development of high blood pressure even after many years. This is certainly a good reason to keep the level of vitamin D in your body very high.

Thankfully, vitamin D is not only available from the sun, because what the body absorbs from the sun is not enough. There are supplements that give you direct vitamin D, which the body needs to help reduce the risk of developing blood pressure.

## 18. Vitamin D Can Also Help Obese Persons

If you are obese or overweight, you will definitely need more vitamin D than someone who is slim.

This is also applicable to those who have a higher body weight, because of their muscle mass.

The most ideal way to get vitamin D for this purpose is through exposure to sunlight without any use of sunblock on the skin.

It is the more natural way to optimize your vitamin D levels. The most ideal time to get the most out of this type of vitamin D is between 9:00 am and 1:00 pm during the day.

## 19. To Reap More Benefits, Get the Best Form of Vitamin D Safely

It has been explained that the ultraviolet light from the sun presents the best source of vitamin D. However, is may not be possible to get enough of the sunlight source of vitamin D because of changing weather conditions throughout the year.

Also, too much exposure to the sun may lead to skin damage, although this depends on your skin type and geographical location.

If you live in an area where you don't see sunlight much, the next best alternative would be to make use of a safe tanning bed with electronic ballast.

Please make sure you don't make use of tanning beds that are made of magnetic ballasts. This will even lead to more exposure to the EMF fields. But if you would rather feel safer, knowing you don't stand a risk of burning your skin, there are other options to optimize vitamin D in your body.

Certain kinds of foods such as mushroom and egg yolk are rich in vitamin D. You can also take supplements to improve your vitamin D levels, but you need to be very careful with the dosage to prevent any form of side effects due to over dosage.

## 20. Can Vitamin D Prevent Heart Disease?

Heart disease is the major cause of death in the United States. Research has proven that vitamin D plays its own part in preventing heart disease.

Just like other muscles, the heart muscle can be weakened when the muscle does not build properly.

In addition, vitamin D protects the blood vessels from damage, suppresses the inflammation of the artery, and equally helps to maintain blood pressure. This is why vitamin D is inversely associated with high blood pressure, strokes, and heart attacks.

## 21. Reduction of Tension and Stress

It has been discovered that vitamin D reduces tension and stress. It also helps to reduce pain and body aches by reducing muscle spasms.

Since it helps in cell differentiation and reduces respiratory infections, it therefore ensures that the pain and tension experienced in such conditions are minimized.

## 22. Increase Inhibitory Effects

Melanoma is a persistent vitamin deficiency caused by complete avoidance of the direct exposure to the sun.

In fact, annual premature deaths as a result of excessive UV exposure have increased over the years as a result of people's tendency to form protective shields against the direct exposure to the sun, which leads to vitamin D deficiency.

This definitely makes sense given that the cancers that are particularly related to vitamin D deficiency are breast, prostate, and colorectal cancer, which are some of the deadliest types of cancers in the United States.

## 23. It Improves Cardiovascular Health

Vitamin D also has close ties with cardiovascular health. Statistics show that deaths from cardiovascular disease fit geographical and seasonal variation, which implies strongly that inadequate sun exposure is a main factor.

Increased parathyroid levels are bound to develop into cardiovascular disease, and fortunately vitamin D minimizes serum parathyroid levels. Lack of vitamin D is also linked with an increased risk of other cardiovascular diseases such as rheumatoid arthritis, Alzheimer's disease, autism, and multiple sclerosis.

## 24. Its Role in Improving the Central Nervous System

The human central nervous system consists of the brain and spinal cord. These lie in the midline of the body and are protected by the skull and vertebrae respectively.

The spinal extensions of the CNS affect body organs and skeletal muscles while the neurons of the CNS affect mental activity and consciousness.

Vitamin D plays a major role here because it supplies calcitriol to body tissues, including the ones in the CNS, helping it to function effectively.

## 25. Helps to Promote Healthy Kidneys

The kidney remains a very integral organ in the body. There is evidence that suggests that vitamin D3 helps to maintain good healthy kidneys.

To understand how this is possible, here is a breakdown of how vitamin D is taken into the body: it is absorbed by the skin through the sun, makes its way to the liver, where it is then transformed into hydroxyvitamin D (calcidio), which is the form that is most accurately measured and found during a blood test.

From the liver, the vitamin then finds its way to the kidney where it is absorbed and converted into dihydroxy-vitamin D (or calcitriol). This form of vitamin D is the most active in the body and is also that circulates to every body tissue.

## 26. Vitamin D and Mortality

With all these benefits of vitamin D, it shouldn't be hard to understand that vitamin D can extend one's life expectancy.

For further proof, there was a systematic review in 2011 conducted from more than 50 studies that looked at more than 80,000 people to establish a correlation between vitamin D and life expectancy.

The research involved elderly women who were given vitamin D3 supplements for a period of 6 months. They found out that their health improved drastically within the period they were on D3 compared to when they had not been given any supplements.

## 27. It is Involved in the Treatment of Uncontrolled Asthma

There are some asthma types that may not respond to normal treatment for the disease.

Researchers discovered that vitamin D reduces the molecular IL-17A level—a substance produced by cells from asthma patients. This molecule is known to have a bearing from an abnormal immune response. Vitamin D comes into play here as it helps keep a proper balance in the immune reaction.

## 28. Choosing the Right Amount of Vitamin D Will Help Prevent Complications

We have seen the overall and specific benefits of vitamin D, but despite all this, it is not advisable to walk into a nutrition store and just order any type of vitamin D supplement you want.

You have to choose wisely because taking the wrong one might cause more harm than good. Vitamins D2 and D3 are the most common types of vitamin D available as a supplement.

But D3 provides more benefits than its closest alternative. D3 is known to raise more vitamin D3 levels in people than other forms of vitamin D.

If you're enjoying this book and would love to let other potential readers know how great it is, please take a few seconds to leave a review on Amazon.com.

## Chapter 4

# What Happens to People Who Have Vitamin D Deficiency?

The knowledge society has on the benefits of vitamin D today is a result of constant research on the complications that come from people who lack enough vitamin D in their body.

Low levels of vitamin D cause a lot of complications, such as rickets among children and osteomalacia in adults. This disease is more common in the developing world than in the developed world. Nevertheless, vitamin D deficiency is really a global concern in old people, as it leads to bone damage and impaired bone mineralization.

## Lack of it May Also Lead to Osteomalacia

This usually occurs in adults. It is characterized by softening of the bone, which leads to bone fragility, proximal muscle weakness, bowing of the legs, bending of the spine, softening of the bone, and a higher risk of fractures. This condition reduces the absorption of calcium and increase the loss of calcium in the bone.

## Vitamin D Deficiency May Cause Rickets

Rickets is a disease most common among children that results in weak and deformed long bones. Children who have rickets have bow legs when they are walking. The primary causes of this condition are, a deficiency in calcium and vitamin D. It is most commonly seen in low income countries and in children with genetic disorders like pseudovitamin D deficiency.

Pregnant women who have little exposure to the sun and who do not have a high amount of vitamin D in their body also stand the risk of transferring this condition to their children when they eventually give birth.

So, vitamin D may be needed more by pregnant women than other classes of people.

# Discover Scientifically-Proven "Shortcuts" & "Hacks" to Lose Weight FASTER (With Very Little Effort)

For this month only, you can get Linda's best-selling & most popular book absolutely free – *Weight Loss Secrets You NEED to Know*.

Get Your FREE Copy Here:
**TopFitnessAdvice.com/Bonus**

Discover scientifically-proven tips to help you lose weight faster and easier than ever before. With this book, readers were able to improve their weight loss results and fitness levels. So, it's highly recommended that you get this book, especially while it's free!

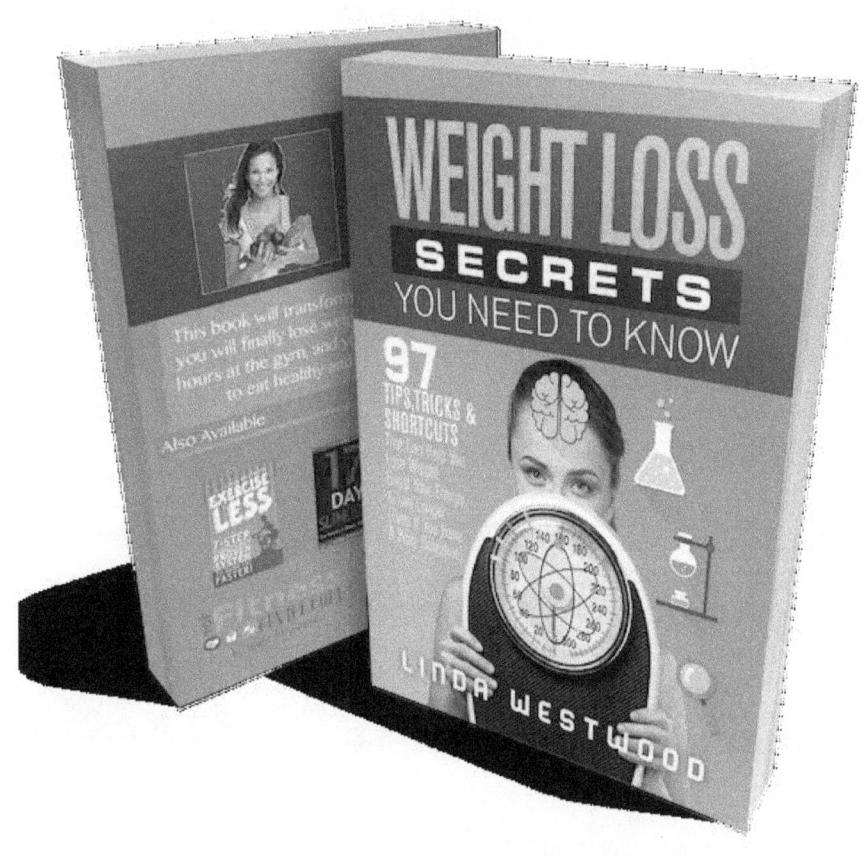

Get Your FREE Copy Here:

**TopFitnessAdvice.com/Bonus**

# Conclusion

Vitamin D is not just a vitamin, it's also a hormone that plays a great role in a wide range of body processes. There has been a lot of research in the last two decades on the benefits of vitamin D in the proper functioning of the body.

Remarkably, this vitamin has been found in about 40 different tissues in the body, including the brain, immune-system cells, muscle, pancreas, and the heart.

So, when it comes to dealing with complications such as diabetes, high blood pressure, cancer, heart disease, and even the common cold, vitamin D has proved to be of vital use to ward off these life-threatening diseases. Furthermore, the sunshine vitamin, as it is usually called, can help you maintain your body weight and prevent you from getting overweight.

This is because the vitamin produces leptin, a hormone that reduces your appetite for food. Similarly, vitamin D also leads to insulin resistance, which would result to greater appetite and overeating if it's not resisted.

The importance of vitamin D to proper functioning of the body cannot be emphasized enough.

There is a need therefore to always maintain an optimum level of this vitamin in the body through sunlight, vitamin-rich foods, and supplements to energize you and help you stay healthy at all times.

Don't forget to share your thoughts on this book by leaving a review on Amazon.com. It takes just a few seconds.

# Final Words

I would like to thank you for purchasing my book and I hope I have been able to help you and educate you on something new.

**If you have enjoyed this book and would like to share your positive thoughts, could you please take 30 seconds of your time to go back and give me a review on my Amazon book page.**

**I greatly appreciate seeing these reviews because it helps me share my hard work.**

You can leave me a review on Amazon.com.

Again, thank you and I wish you all the best!

# Enjoying this book?

# Check out my other best sellers!

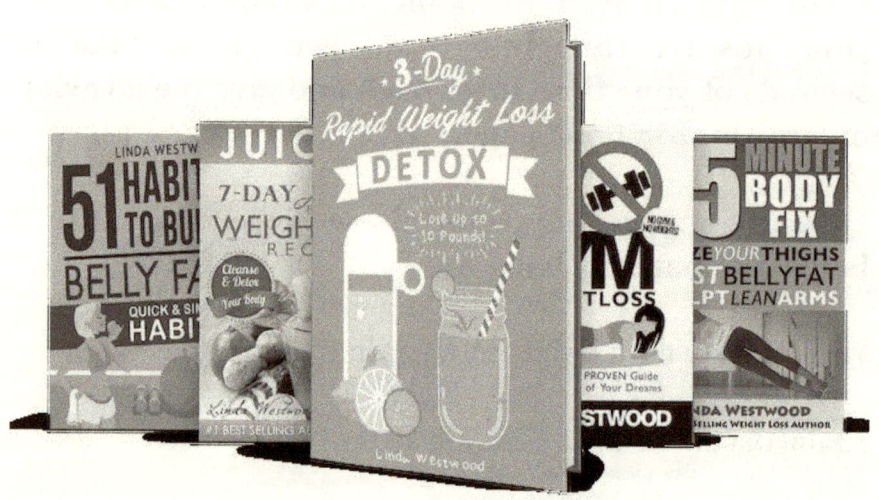

Get your next book on sale here:

TopFitnessAdvice.com/go/books

www.ingramcontent.com/pod-product-compliance
Lightning Source LLC
Chambersburg PA
CBHW031209020426
42333CB00013B/863